SKIN RADIANCE RITUALS

Therapies For A Youthful And Glowing Complexion

Achieve Radiant Skin Through A Series Of Therapeutic Rituals Designed To Promote Skin Health And Vitality

DR. BRIDGET PROMISE

Table of Contents

CHAPTER ONE

Introduction

Many people have the urge to have bright, beautiful skin, and this desire often extends beyond aesthetics. Gaining this desired complexion requires first knowing the science behind skin brightness. Bright, healthy skin is a sign of general well-being.

This path entails embracing a thorough skincare regimen, beginning with the fundamentals and adding regular rituals that address the particular requirements of your skin. Effective cleaning is essential to this quest since it holds the key to uncovering the secrets of glowing skin. We explore the science of skin brightness in this inquiry, start with the fundamentals of skincare, and walk you through your daily morning and nighttime routines—with a particular emphasis on the art of efficient washing.

Knowing The Science Behind Skin Radiance

The skin is the biggest organ in the human body, and a wide range of variables affect both its look and health. It's common to equate radiant skin with attributes like natural radiance, moisture, and even tone. To understand the science behind radiant skin, one must investigate the physiological factors that lead to a bright complexion.

Collagen, a protein that gives the skin its structural support, is one important component. Collagen prevents wrinkles and sagging by maintaining the skin's elasticity and firmness. Visible indications of aging result from a natural decline in collagen formation as we age. A more radiant complexion may be achieved by using skincare techniques that encourage the manufacture of collagen, such as utilizing products containing retinoids or peptides.

Hydration is another important factor in radiant skin. Dehydrated skin lacks the brightness and dreary appearance of healthy skin. Maintaining the skin's moisture balance and looking beautiful are made possible by consuming a sufficient quantity of water and hydrating skincare products.

Knowing your skin type is also very important. Every skin type has different requirements, and you may improve the radiance of your skin by utilizing products designed for your particular kind. People with oily skin, for example, can benefit from mattifying, oil-free products, whilst people with dry skin would need heavier formulas to seal in moisture.

The Basis: Skincare Essentials For A Radiant Complexion

Learning the fundamentals of skincare is the first step in creating a strong foundation for attractive skin. This calls for a few basic actions that have to be a part of your everyday regimen, both in the morning and at night.

1. Cleaning: A good cleaning regimen is the foundation of any skincare regimen. In this stage, pollutants, oil, and filth that build up on the skin during the day are removed. To prevent removing natural oils from your skin, which may cause dullness and dryness, use a mild cleanser that is appropriate for your skin type.

2. Exfoliation: Dead skin cells may build up on the skin's surface and make it seem dull. Regular exfoliation is key to removing these cells. Use a light exfoliation on your skin two to three times a week to encourage cell turnover and reveal bright, new skin.

3. Moisturizing: Having hydrated skin is essential to having glowing skin. By putting on a moisturizer, you may help seal in moisture and provide a barrier that protects against environmental irritants. Whether it's a thicker cream for dry skin or a lighter gel for oily skin, choose a moisturizer that works for your skin type.

4. Sunscreen: You must shield your skin from the damaging effects of ultraviolet light. Even on gloomy days, sunscreen should be worn in the morning to avoid sunspots, premature aging, and other skin conditions that may reduce radiance.

Morning and Nighttime Rituals: A Bright Skincare Program

When it comes to skincare, routines should be followed religiously. Creating morning and nighttime rituals may help you achieve and keep glowing skin.

Morning Schedule

1. Cleaning: To get rid of any pollutants that could have been collected overnight, start your day with a mild cleaner.

2. Toning: Use a toner to bring your skin's pH levels back into equilibrium and get it ready for the next stages.

3. Serum: To shield your skin from environmental harm and encourage the production of collagen, use a serum that contains antioxidants, such as vitamin C.

4. Moisturizer: Use a moisturizer that is appropriate for your skin type to seal in moisture.

5. Sunscreen: To protect your skin from UV radiation, use a broad-spectrum sunscreen after your morning routine.

Evening Schedule:

1. Cleaning: To get rid of the accumulation from the day,

remove your makeup and give your skin a good cleansing.

2. Exfoliation: To encourage cell turnover, including exfoliation in your evening regimen.

3. Treatment: To get the most out of any targeted therapies you employ, such as serums or retinoids, use them at night.

4. Apply a little layer of eye cream to target particular issues such as fine lines or dark circles.

5. Moisturizer: To help your skin heal while you sleep, seal in moisture with a nutritious night cream or moisturizer.

CHAPTER TWO

Cracking The Code Of Successful Cleaning

Cleaning is an art that bears the secret to glowing skin, not merely a preemptive measure. Understanding your skin's requirements and selecting the appropriate products and methods are essential to effective washing.

1. Select the Correct Cleanser: Various skin types need distinct cleansers. To manage excess oil on your oily skin, use a foamy or gel-based cleanser. Select a

moisturizing cleanser for dry skin that doesn't remove vital moisture.

2. Double Cleaning: Take into account using the double cleaning technique, particularly at night. To remove sunscreen and makeup, start with an oil-based cleanser and finish with a water-based cleanser to leave the skin feeling clean.

3. Gentle Cleaning Methods: Treat your skin gently, particularly in the vicinity of your sensitive eye region. Instead of using abrasive scrubbing that might irritate the skin, use your fingers or a gentle cloth to clean.

4.	Maintaining	Consistency:
Cleanse your skin often, but don't go overboard. Over-cleansing and the use of strong treatments may damage the skin's protective layer, causing dryness and irritation.

5. Seasonally Adjust: The demands placed on your skin might vary depending on the season. You may require a more moisturizing cleanser in the winter, but in the summer, a lighter one can be good enough.

To sum up, achieving beautiful skin requires a mix of comprehending the science behind it, building a strong foundation with skincare essentials, and implementing daily routines that are tailored to your skin's specific requirements. Unlocking the keys to glowing skin, in particular, requires effective cleaning to make sure your complexion shines with health and vigor.

You may start a transformational path towards having the radiant skin you want by accepting these concepts and customizing them to your skin type.

Exfoliation Methods For Skin That Is Smoother And Brighter

Everyone wants to have glowing, smooth skin, and one of the most important first steps in getting there is exfoliation. By removing dead skin cells from the skin's surface, this skincare method reveals a complexion that is more vivid and fresh. Different exfoliation techniques are available, each addressing distinct skin types and issues.

Using granular materials like sugar or microbeads in a scrub to physically slough off dead skin cells is known as physical exfoliation. This technique works well to improve the texture of the skin and encourage cell turnover. To prevent irritation and harm to the skin barrier, physical exfoliation must be done gently.

In contrast, chemical exfoliation dissolves dead skin cells by using acids such as beta hydroxy acids (BHAs) or alpha hydroxy acids (AHAs). AHAs that operate on the skin's surface, such as lactic and glycolic acid, enhance texture and encourage a glowing complexion. Because BHAs like salicylic acid get deeper into the pores, they are especially beneficial for those with oily or acne-prone skin.

It's crucial to find the ideal balance for exfoliation. Excessive exfoliating may exacerbate some skin issues and cause redness and irritation. Depending on your skin type and the product you use, exfoliating one to three times a week is advised.

Heroes Of Hydration: The Potency Of Moisturizing

Regardless of your skin type, the first step in any skincare regimen is always to moisturize. It is essential for preserving the health of the skin since it keeps the skin hydrated and strengthens its natural barrier of defense. A moisturized skin barrier is more resilient to aggressors from the outside and maintains its young, supple look.

The best moisturizer for each person's skin type will vary. Choose a thick, emollient cream that offers great hydration if you have dry skin. Oil-free, non-comedogenic formulations that regulate moisture without blocking pores are beneficial for oily or acne-prone skin. For mixed skin, gel-based moisturizers are a great option since they provide moisture without being too oily.

The application technique is just as important as choosing the appropriate product. Moisturizers work better at retaining moisture when applied to wet skin. Patting the substance into the skin as opposed to rubbing it in lessens the chance of irritation and decreases friction.

CHAPTER THREE

Targeted Luminosity Treatments Using Serums And Elixirs

Concentrated formulas called serums and elixirs are designed to address certain skin issues and provide strong active ingredients. These products are perfect for stacking in a skincare regimen since they are lightweight and readily absorbed.

Adding serums and elixirs to your routine may help with fine wrinkles, hyperpigmentation, dullness, and other issues.

Brightening qualities are well known for vitamin C serums. They balance out skin tone, reduce the appearance of dark spots, and provide antioxidant defense against environmental deterioration. Hydrating powerhouses, hyaluronic acid serums draw and hold moisture for plump, glossy skin. Vitamin A-based retinol serums increase cell turnover, which minimizes the visibility of fine lines and encourages a smoother complexion.

To make sure a serum is compatible with your skin type, patch test it before adding it to your regimen. To avoid any possible irritation and to keep an eye on its effects, introduce one new product at a time.

Sunscreen: Your Protective Layer Against Early Aging

An essential component of any skincare regimen is sunscreen. One of the main factors causing early aging is exposure to ultraviolet (UV) radiation, which also causes wrinkles, fine lines, and hyperpigmentation. It is recommended to use a broad-spectrum sunscreen with a minimum SPF of 30 every day, even on overcast days or in the winter.

UVA and UVB are the two damaging radiation kinds that the sun generates. While UVB rays induce sunburn, UVA rays deeply enter the skin and cause premature aging. Broad-spectrum sunscreens provide complete protection from both kinds of radiation.

It's important to apply sunscreen consistently. Apply it liberally on the face, neck, hands, and any other exposed skin areas. Every two hours, or more often if swimming or perspiring, reapplication is required. Sunscreen is a crucial component of skin health maintenance since it not only reduces the risk of skin cancer but also prevents premature aging.

Eating From The Inside Out: How Nutrition Affects Skin Brightness

Although exterior skincare regimens are important, interior aspects like food also play a significant impact. In terms of skin health, the adage "you are what you eat" is accurate. A complexion full of vitamins, minerals, and antioxidants may be achieved with a well-balanced diet.

Foods high in antioxidants, such as citrus fruits, leafy greens, and berries, fight free radicals, which cause aging and skin damage. Walnuts, flaxseeds, and fatty fish are good sources of omega-3 fatty acids, which help keep skin supple and moisturized. Vitamin C helps produce collagen, which promotes firmness and elasticity. It is found in abundance in oranges, strawberries, and bell peppers.

For healthy skin, staying hydrated is equally important. By keeping the skin clean and moisturized from the inside out, drinking enough water aids in the removal of toxins. Reducing alcohol, processed food, and sugar intake may also help you have a healthy complexion.

In summary, a comprehensive strategy that incorporates efficient exfoliation, enough hydration, targeted treatments, sun protection, and a healthy diet is necessary to achieve smoother, brighter, and more radiant skin. People may discover the keys to a radiant and young complexion by including these techniques in a regular skincare regimen.

Maximizing Overnight Skin Repair With Beauty Sleep

Not only is "beauty sleep" a catchy word, but it also has scientific validity. Good sleep has a major influence on skin health and is essential for general wellness. The body, including the skin, enters into repair mode while you sleep.

Deep sleep is when the most collagen, a protein necessary for skin suppleness, is produced. Insufficient sleep has been linked to elevated stress levels, which may trigger the production of cortisol, a hormone that has the potential to degrade collagen. Wrinkles, fine lines, and premature aging may be caused by this collagen degradation.

It's crucial to give good sleep a top priority if you want to optimize overnight skin restoration. Try to get between seven and nine hours of sleep every night.

Create a peaceful sleeping environment, stick to a regular sleep schedule, and stay away from stimulants like coffee just before bed.

CHAPTER FOUR

Homemade Face Masks For Bright And Revitalised Skin

Self-care activities, like making homemade face masks, maybe a relaxing approach to reduce stress and encourage glowing, refreshed skin. Natural nutrients that can nourish and regenerate the skin include avocado, yogurt, honey, and turmeric.

For instance, turmeric has anti-inflammatory and brightening qualities, while honey is recognized for its moisturizing and antibacterial qualities.

Making your DIY face mask is easy and customizable to suit your skin type. Yogurt and turmeric may be used in a brightening mask, while avocado and honey might used in a moisturizing mask. In addition to offering noticeable beauty benefits, these masks give a meditative and soothing experience that helps lower stress levels.

Including homemade face masks regularly in your skincare regimen gives you a chance to take a break from everyday concerns and prioritize self-care. A comprehensive approach to stress management for young skin will benefit greatly from the enjoyable addition of these masks, whether they are used as a weekly routine or an occasional pleasure.

Gua Sha And Facial Massage: Traditional Methods For Contemporary Radiance

Ancient Chinese medical treatments like gua sha and face massage have become more and more popular in contemporary skincare regimens. Gua Sha promotes lymphatic drainage and reduces puffiness by gently massaging and scraping the skin with an instrument with a smooth edge. On the other hand, a facial massage uses specialized equipment or the hands to knead and activate the muscles of the face.

These methods may greatly improve the skin's look and health in addition to providing relaxation. Facial massage and Gua Sha both improve blood circulation and lymphatic drainage, which contributes to a healthy glow. Additionally, it may be possible to prevent or lessen the appearance of wrinkles and fine lines by stimulating the muscles in the face.

Including these age-old methods in your skincare regimen may be a comprehensive strategy for managing stress. In addition to relieving physical strain, the rhythmic and focused practices of Gua Sha and face massage also provide a psychological and emotional boost. You may promote the health of your skin and your general well-being by including these practices in your regimen daily.

Including Face Yoga In Your Everyday Routine

A series of movements known as "facial yoga" are intended to target and tone the muscles in the face and neck. Facial yoga has acquired popularity despite its original strange seeming notion due to its possible advantages in promoting a young look. The workouts include a variety of motions, including massages, stretches for the face, and strength training for the face's muscles.

These workouts are designed to enhance muscular tone, promote collagen synthesis, and improve blood circulation. Facial yoga is a thoughtful activity that may help reduce stress, and it can also improve the general health and look of your skin when you include it in your daily routine.

It is simple to include facial yoga poses into skincare regimens already in place or to do them on their own. It might be as little as five to ten minutes a day. The secret is to be consistent since long-term effects need consistent practice. These exercises, which include the "lion face" and "cheek lifter," may help you reduce stress and enjoyably maintain toned, young skin.

To sum up, comprehensive methods of stress reduction are essential for keeping skin looking young and glowing. Facial yoga, Gua Sha, beauty sleep, facial massage, and DIY face masks are all parts of a holistic approach that tackles stress's emotional and physical components. By adopting these routines, you may promote general well-being in a comprehensive and long-lasting way, in addition to improving the health and beauty of your skin.

Natural Treatments For Typical Skin Issues

Many people go to different skincare products that promise revolutionary results in their quest for healthy, glowing skin. On the other hand, adopting a natural skincare regimen may be both mild and effective. You may design an individualized skincare regimen that promotes well-being and targets certain problems by learning about common skin disorders and combining natural therapies relevant to your skin type.

CHAPTER FIVE

Developing A Skincare Program Specific To Your Skin Type

Understanding and identifying your skin type is one of the cornerstones of good skincare. Different skin types have different demands, and you may get better results if you customize your regimen to meet these needs. The four primary varieties of skin are combination, oily, dry, and sensitive.

Using natural solutions for oily skin, including witch hazel or tea tree oil, may help reduce excessive sebum production. These natural astringent qualities of the substances prevent oiliness without depriving the skin of vital moisture.

Conversely, moisturizing substances like aloe vera, honey, or olive oil are beneficial for dry skin. Deep hydration is offered by these organic moisturizers, which also help to regulate the skin's natural moisture levels and soothe dry areas.

Combination skin needs a well-rounded strategy that addresses many issues in distinct regions. Rose water or chamomile are two examples of components that may be used to keep things in balance while also reducing oiliness and relieving dryness.

Calendula, chamomile, and cucumber are popular natural treatments for their relaxing and soothing qualities, which are ideal for sensitive skin that needs additional care. For those with sensitive skin, staying away from strong chemicals and scents is essential; choosing mild, natural components may help avoid discomfort.

The Practice Of Conscious Skincare: Developing Self-Care Routines

Skincare is a chance to exercise mindfulness and self-care, not just a routine. Your whole well-being may benefit from setting aside some time each day to practice mindful skincare and establish a connection with your skin.

Establish a calm space for your skincare routine first. Take advantage of this time to relax and permit yourself to let go of your worries from the day. From cleaning to applying treatments, be mindful of every step and savor the feeling of taking care of yourself.

Being aware of your skin's requirements is another aspect of mindful skincare. Take note of how various products affect your skin's response and modify your regimen appropriately. This awareness fosters a closer relationship with oneself by enabling you to make knowledgeable choices about what is best for your skin.

Sustaining Glory Throughout Various Life Stages

Our skin changes throughout our lives due to a variety of variables, including hormones, age, and environment. Maintaining brightness across various life phases requires you to modify your skincare regimen to fit your skin's changing demands.

In your twenties, concentrate on building a solid skincare regimen. Put antioxidants like vitamin C first to defend against environmental stresses. This helps prevent early indications of aging in addition to protecting your skin.

As you approach your thirties and forties, think about adding collagen-stimulating treatments like retinol. This may help maintain skin suppleness and lessen the look of fine wrinkles.

Hydration becomes critical for those in their fifties and beyond. To counteract the consequences of decreased skin elasticity and moisture retention, invest in nourishing, rich moisturizers and serums. Accept the knowledge of growing older with elegance and treasure the distinct beauty that emerges with every year that passes.

Dispelling Often Held Myths And Misconceptions About Skincare

Knowing what is true and what is fiction in the huge world of skincare advice is essential. Frequently held beliefs and misunderstandings may cause you to follow incorrect habits and even damage your skin. Let's bust some common misconceptions about skincare.

Myth 1: "Natural means safe for all skin types." Although natural products have their advantages, it's important to keep in mind that each person has different allergies and sensitivities. To prevent negative responses, it is essential to patch-test new goods and chemicals.

Myth 2: "Daily exfoliation results in smoother skin." Exfoliation is good, but too much of it may remove the skin's protective layer, which can cause sensitivity and inflammation. Choose products with mild exfoliants, such as fruit acids or jojoba beads, and limit your weekly exfoliation to two or three times.

Myth 3: "Sunscreen is only needed on sunny days." UV radiation can penetrate clouds as well, so wearing sunscreen every day is essential to preventing skin cancer and premature aging. Apply sunscreen regularly, no matter the weather.

In Summary

The path to glowing, healthy skin is quite individualized in the world of skincare. Achieving optimum skin health involves embracing natural therapies according to your skin type, developing a thoughtful skincare regimen, adjusting to your skin's changing demands as you go through various life phases, and busting common misconceptions.

By being aware of the special qualities of your skin and using a holistic skincare regimen, you may improve the outside appearance of your appearance while also fostering a closer relationship with yourself. Keep in mind that skincare is a self-care ritual that enables you to enjoy and value the skin you're in at every stage of life, not just a regimen.

www.ingramcontent.com/pod-product-compliance
Lightning Source LLC
Chambersburg PA
CBHW071121260726
48661CB00006B/2670